THE ONE-MINUTE GRATITUDE JOURNAL FOR MEN

SIMPLE JOURNAL TO INCREASE GRATITUDE AND HAPPINESS

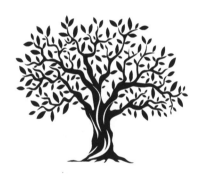

This Journal belongs to:

_____

ISBN: 978-1-952358-25-8

Gratitude

Gratitude is a feeling of appreciation for what one has. It is a feeling of thankfulness for the blessings we have received. Cultivating an attitude of gratitude yields many benefits: physical, mental and spiritual. Feeling gratitude in the present moment makes you happier and more relaxed, and improves your overall health and well-being.

With an eye made quiet by the power of harmony, and the deep power of joy,
we see into the life of things.
~ William Wordsworth

Gratitude doesn't just have to be about the big things. It can also be for small, everyday events. You can be thankful for simple things such as enjoying a movie or just talking to an old friend for the first time in a long while. There is always something that you can be grateful for in your life. It is all about appreciating the things around you rather than taking them all for granted.

Write down three to five things that you are grateful for each day. You will not only feel good as you write them down, but you will experience gratitude during the day as well. A person experiencing gratitude feels a sense of joy and abundance in their life. They also feel more connected with other people and have increased energy.

Gratitude should always be expressed in the present tense and is more powerful when combined with the perceived benefit so that an emotional connection is made. Instead of writing, *"I am grateful for my health and well-being,"* it is better to write, *"I am grateful for my health and well-being and it makes me feel great."*

No duty is more urgent than that of returning thanks.
~ James Allen

One of the healthiest and most positive things we can do in our lives is to express our gratitude to the people around us. Tell someone how much you appreciate them. Tell someone that something they did mattered to you. When people make an impact, let them know. We are usually too quick to point out people's faults and ways in which they have wronged us, while slow to bestow recognition for good deeds and favors.

If someone makes you feel good, make them feel good too. By expressing our gratitude to others, we are making the world a better place and encouraging the things that we want to see more of. Say, *"Thank you."* Make a difference. Seek out the best in people and when you find it, say something about it.

A gentle word, a kind look, a good-natured smile can work wonders and accomplish miracles.
~ William Hazlitt

Gratitude makes us more optimistic and compassionate. True happiness lies within us. By keeping a record of your gratitude in a journal, you will store positive energy, gain clarity in your life, and have greater control of your thoughts and emotions.

Each day, write down three to five things that you are grateful for in this journal and turn your ordinary moments into blessings.

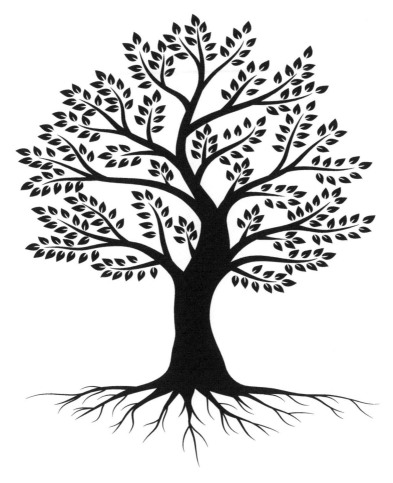

A contented mind is the greatest blessing a man can enjoy in this world.

~ Joseph Addison

Happiness is not an ideal of reason, but of imagination.
— Immanuel Kant

Day: _____   Date: _/_/___

1. Today I am *Grateful* for:

_____

_____

_____

_____

_____

2. What's one thing you can do to make today great?

_____

Day: _____   Date: _/_/___

1. Today I am *Grateful* for:

_____

_____

_____

_____

_____

2. What's one thing you can do to make today great?

_____

Day: _____   Date: _/_/___

1. Today I am *Grateful* for:

_____

_____

_____

_____

_____

2. What's one thing you can do to make today great?

_____

Three grand essentials to happiness in this life are something to do, something to love, and something to hope for. — Joseph Addison

Day: _____   Date: __/__/___

1. Today I am *Grateful* for:

_____

_____

_____

_____

_____

2. What's one thing you can do to make today great?

_____

Day: _____   Date: __/__/___

1. Today I am *Grateful* for:

_____

_____

_____

_____

_____

2. What's one thing you can do to make today great?

_____

Day: _____   Date: __/__/___

1. Today I am *Grateful* for:

_____

_____

_____

_____

2. What's one thing you can do to make today great?

_____

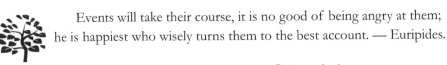

Events will take their course, it is no good of being angry at them; he is happiest who wisely turns them to the best account. — Euripides.

Day: _____   Date: __/__/____

1. Today I am *Grateful* for:

_____

_____

_____

_____

_____

2. What's one thing you can do to make today great?

_____

Day: _____   Date: __/__/____

1. Today I am *Grateful* for:

_____

_____

_____

_____

_____

2. What's one thing you can do to make today great?

_____

Day: _____   Date: __/__/____

1. Today I am *Grateful* for:

_____

_____

_____

_____

_____

2. What's one thing you can do to make today great?

_____

Our life is what our thoughts make it.
— Marcus Aurelius

Day: _____   Date: __/__/____

1. Today I am *Grateful* for:

_____

_____

_____

_____

_____

2. What's one thing you can do to make today great?

_____

Day: _____   Date: __/__/____

1. Today I am *Grateful* for:

_____

_____

_____

_____

_____

2. What's one thing you can do to make today great?

_____

Day: _____   Date: __/__/____

1. Today I am *Grateful* for:

_____

_____

_____

_____

_____

2. What's one thing you can do to make today great?

_____

Write it on your heart that every day is the best day in the year.
— Ralph Waldo Emerson

Day: _____   Date: __/__/___

1. Today I am *Grateful* for:

_____

_____

_____

_____

_____

2. What's one thing you can do to make today great?

_____

Day: _____   Date: __/__/___

1. Today I am *Grateful* for:

_____

_____

_____

_____

_____

2. What's one thing you can do to make today great?

_____

Day: _____   Date: __/__/___

1. Today I am *Grateful* for:

_____

_____

_____

_____

_____

2. What's one thing you can do to make today great?

_____

Our greatest weakness lies in giving up. The most certain way to succeed is always to try just one more time. — Thomas A. Edison

Day: _____   Date: __/__/____

1. Today I am *Grateful* for:

_____

_____

_____

_____

_____

2. What's one thing you can do to make today great?

_____

Day: _____   Date: __/__/____

1. Today I am *Grateful* for:

_____

_____

_____

_____

_____

2. What's one thing you can do to make today great?

_____

Day: _____   Date: __/__/____

1. Today I am *Grateful* for:

_____

_____

_____

_____

_____

2. What's one thing you can do to make today great?

_____

It is great happiness to be praised of them who are
most praiseworthy. — Philip Sidney

Day: _____   Date: __/__/____

1. Today I am *Grateful* for:

_____

_____

_____

_____

_____

2. What's one thing you can do to make today great?

_____

Day: _____   Date: __/__/____

1. Today I am *Grateful* for:

_____

_____

_____

_____

_____

2. What's one thing you can do to make today great?

_____

Day: _____   Date: __/__/____

1. Today I am *Grateful* for:

_____

_____

_____

_____

_____

2. What's one thing you can do to make today great?

_____

Our happiness depends on wisdom all the way.
— Sophocles

Day: _____   Date: __/__/____

1. Today I am *Grateful* for:

_____

_____

_____

_____

_____

2. What's one thing you can do to make today great?

_____

Day: _____   Date: __/__/____

1. Today I am *Grateful* for:

_____

_____

_____

_____

_____

2. What's one thing you can do to make today great?

_____

Day: _____   Date: __/__/____

1. Today I am *Grateful* for:

_____

_____

_____

_____

_____

2. What's one thing you can do to make today great?

_____

By appreciation, we make excellence in others our own property.
— Voltaire

Day: _____   Date: __/__/___

1. Today I am *Grateful* for:

_____

_____

_____

_____

_____

2. What's one thing you can do to make today great?

_____

Day: _____   Date: __/__/___

1. Today I am *Grateful* for:

_____

_____

_____

_____

_____

2. What's one thing you can do to make today great?

_____

Day: _____   Date: __/__/___

1. Today I am *Grateful* for:

_____

_____

_____

_____

_____

2. What's one thing you can do to make today great?

_____

The sun does not shine for a few trees and flowers, but for the wide world's joy. — Henry Ward Beecher

Day: _____   Date: __/__/____

1. Today I am *Grateful* for:

_____

_____

_____

_____

_____

2. What's one thing you can do to make today great?

_____

Day: _____   Date: __/__/____

1. Today I am *Grateful* for:

_____

_____

_____

_____

_____

2. What's one thing you can do to make today great?

_____

Day: _____   Date: __/__/____

1. Today I am *Grateful* for:

_____

_____

_____

_____

_____

2. What's one thing you can do to make today great?

_____

Blessed is the influence of one true, loving human soul on another.
— George Eliot

Day: _____   Date: __/__/____

1. Today I am *Grateful* for:

_____

_____

_____

_____

_____

2. What's one thing you can do to make today great?

_____

Day: _____   Date: __/__/____

1. Today I am *Grateful* for:

_____

_____

_____

_____

_____

2. What's one thing you can do to make today great?

_____

Day: _____   Date: __/__/____

1. Today I am *Grateful* for:

_____

_____

_____

_____

_____

2. What's one thing you can do to make today great?

_____

Pleasure is none, if not diversified.
— John Donne

Day: _____   Date: __/__/____

1. Today I am *Grateful* for:

_____
_____
_____
_____
_____

2. What's one thing you can do to make today great?

_____

Day: _____   Date: __/__/____

1. Today I am *Grateful* for:

_____
_____
_____
_____
_____

2. What's one thing you can do to make today great?

_____

Day: _____   Date: __/__/____

1. Today I am *Grateful* for:

_____
_____
_____
_____

2. What's one thing you can do to make today great?

_____

Genius is the ability to renew one's emotions in daily experience.
— Paul Cezanne

Day: _____   Date: __/__/____

1. Today I am *Grateful* for:

_____

_____

_____

_____

_____

2. What's one thing you can do to make today great?

_____

Day: _____   Date: __/__/____

1. Today I am *Grateful* for:

_____

_____

_____

_____

_____

2. What's one thing you can do to make today great?

_____

Day: _____   Date: __/__/____

1. Today I am *Grateful* for:

_____

_____

_____

_____

_____

2. What's one thing you can do to make today great?

_____

Courtesies of a small and trivial character are the ones which
strike deepest in the grateful and appreciating heart. — Henry Clay

Day: _____   Date: __/__/____

1. Today I am *Grateful* for:

_____

_____

_____

_____

_____

2. What's one thing you can do to make today great?

_____

Day: _____   Date: __/__/____

1. Today I am *Grateful* for:

_____

_____

_____

_____

_____

2. What's one thing you can do to make today great?

_____

Day: _____   Date: __/__/____

1. Today I am *Grateful* for:

_____

_____

_____

_____

_____

2. What's one thing you can do to make today great?

_____

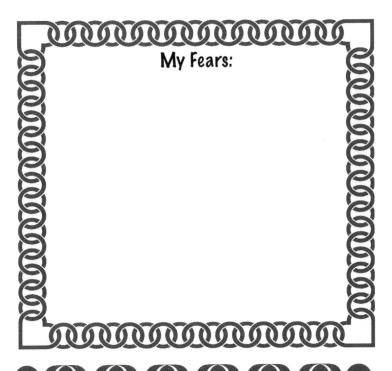

My Fears:

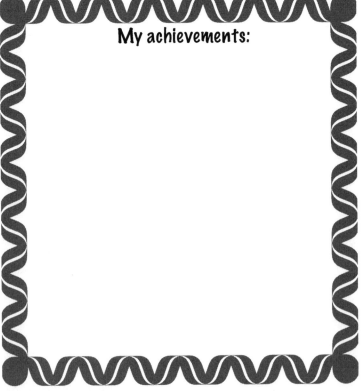

My achievements:

Keep love in your heart. A life without it is like a sunless
garden when the flowers are dead. — Oscar Wilde

Day: _____   Date: __/__/____

1. Today I am *Grateful* for:

_____

_____

_____

_____

_____

_____

2. What's one thing you can do to make today great?

_____

Day: _____   Date: __/__/____

1. Today I am *Grateful* for:

_____

_____

_____

_____

_____

_____

2. What's one thing you can do to make today great?

_____

Day: _____   Date: __/__/____

1. Today I am *Grateful* for:

_____

_____

_____

_____

_____

2. What's one thing you can do to make today great?

_____

Rejoice in the things that are present; all else is beyond thee.
— Michel de Montaigne

Day: _____   Date: __/__/____

1. Today I am *Grateful* for:

_____
_____
_____
_____
_____

2. What's one thing you can do to make today great?

_____

Day: _____   Date: __/__/____

1. Today I am *Grateful* for:

_____
_____
_____
_____
_____

2. What's one thing you can do to make today great?

_____

Day: _____   Date: __/__/____

1. Today I am *Grateful* for:

_____
_____
_____
_____

2. What's one thing you can do to make today great?

_____

By experience we find out a short way by a long wandering.
— Roger Ascham

Day: _____   Date: __/__/____

1. Today I am *Grateful* for:

_____

_____

_____

_____

_____

2. What's one thing you can do to make today great?

_____

Day: _____   Date: __/__/____

1. Today I am *Grateful* for:

_____

_____

_____

_____

_____

2. What's one thing you can do to make today great?

_____

Day: _____   Date: __/__/____

1. Today I am *Grateful* for:

_____

_____

_____

_____

_____

2. What's one thing you can do to make today great?

_____

In character, in manner, in style, in all things, the supreme
excellence is simplicity. — Henry Wadsworth Longfellow

Day: _____   Date: __/__/___

1. Today I am *Grateful* for:

_____

_____

_____

_____

_____

2. What's one thing you can do to make today great?

_____

Day: _____   Date: __/__/___

1. Today I am *Grateful* for:

_____

_____

_____

_____

_____

2. What's one thing you can do to make today great?

_____

Day: _____   Date: __/__/___

1. Today I am *Grateful* for:

_____

_____

_____

_____

_____

2. What's one thing you can do to make today great?

_____

Good means not merely not to do wrong, but rather not to
desire to do wrong. — Democritus

Day: _____ Date: __/__/___

1. Today I am *Grateful* for:

_____
_____
_____
_____
_____

2. What's one thing you can do to make today great?

_____

Day: _____ Date: __/__/___

1. Today I am *Grateful* for:

_____
_____
_____
_____
_____

2. What's one thing you can do to make today great?

_____

Day: _____ Date: __/__/___

1. Today I am *Grateful* for:

_____
_____
_____
_____
_____

2. What's one thing you can do to make today great?

_____

Day: _____   Date: ___/___/____

1. Today I am *Grateful* for:

_____

_____

_____

_____

_____

2. What's one thing you can do to make today great?

_____

Day: _____   Date: ___/___/____

1. Today I am *Grateful* for:

_____

_____

_____

_____

_____

2. What's one thing you can do to make today great?

_____

Day: _____   Date: ___/___/____

1. Today I am *Grateful* for:

_____

_____

_____

_____

_____

2. What's one thing you can do to make today great?

_____

Day: _____   Date: __/__/____

1. Today I am *Grateful* for:

_____

_____

_____

_____

_____

2. What's one thing you can do to make today great?

_____

Day: _____   Date: __/__/____

1. Today I am *Grateful* for:

_____

_____

_____

_____

_____

2. What's one thing you can do to make today great?

_____

Day: _____   Date: __/__/____

1. Today I am *Grateful* for:

_____

_____

_____

_____

_____

2. What's one thing you can do to make today great?

_____

Out of nothing can come, and nothing can become nothing.
— Persius

Day: _____   Date: __/__/____

1. Today I am *Grateful* for:

_____

_____

_____

_____

_____

2. What's one thing you can do to make today great?

_____

Day: _____   Date: __/__/____

1. Today I am *Grateful* for:

_____

_____

_____

_____

_____

2. What's one thing you can do to make today great?

_____

Day: _____   Date: __/__/____

1. Today I am *Grateful* for:

_____

_____

_____

_____

_____

2. What's one thing you can do to make today great?

_____

It is the heart always that sees, before the head can see.
— Thomas Carlyle

Day: _____   Date: __/__/____

1. Today I am *Grateful* for:

_____

_____

_____

_____

_____

2. What's one thing you can do to make today great?

_____

Day: _____   Date: __/__/____

1. Today I am *Grateful* for:

_____

_____

_____

_____

_____

2. What's one thing you can do to make today great?

_____

Day: _____   Date: __/__/____

1. Today I am *Grateful* for:

_____

_____

_____

_____

_____

2. What's one thing you can do to make today great?

_____

The best preparation for tomorrow is to do today's
work superbly well. — William Osler

Day: _____   Date: __/__/___

1. Today I am *Grateful* for:

_____

_____

_____

_____

_____

2. What's one thing you can do to make today great?

_____

Day: _____   Date: __/__/___

1. Today I am *Grateful* for:

_____

_____

_____

_____

_____

2. What's one thing you can do to make today great?

_____

Day: _____   Date: __/__/___

1. Today I am *Grateful* for:

_____

_____

_____

_____

_____

2. What's one thing you can do to make today great?

_____

Good actions give strength to ourselves and inspire good
actions in others. — Plato

Day: _____   Date: __/__/____

1. Today I am *Grateful* for:

_____

_____

_____

_____

_____

2. What's one thing you can do to make today great?

_____

Day: _____   Date: __/__/____

1. Today I am *Grateful* for:

_____

_____

_____

_____

_____

2. What's one thing you can do to make today great?

_____

Day: _____   Date: __/__/____

1. Today I am *Grateful* for:

_____

_____

_____

_____

_____

2. What's one thing you can do to make today great?

_____

Make it your habit not to be critical about small things.
— Edward Everett Hale

Day: _____   Date: __/__/____

1. Today I am *Grateful* for:

_____

_____

_____

_____

_____

2. What's one thing you can do to make today great?

_____

Day: _____   Date: __/__/____

1. Today I am *Grateful* for:

_____

_____

_____

_____

_____

2. What's one thing you can do to make today great?

_____

Day: _____   Date: __/__/____

1. Today I am *Grateful* for:

_____

_____

_____

_____

_____

2. What's one thing you can do to make today great?

_____

Grace is the beauty of form under the influence
of freedom. — Friedrich Schiller

Day: _____   Date: __/__/___

1. Today I am *Grateful* for:

_____

_____

_____

_____

_____

2. What's one thing you can do to make today great?

_____

Day: _____   Date: __/__/___

1. Today I am *Grateful* for:

_____

_____

_____

_____

_____

2. What's one thing you can do to make today great?

_____

Day: _____   Date: __/__/___

1. Today I am *Grateful* for:

_____

_____

_____

_____

_____

2. What's one thing you can do to make today great?

_____

Great works are performed not by strength but by perseverance.
— Samuel Johnson

Day: _____   Date: __/__/___

1. Today I am *Grateful* for:

_____
_____
_____
_____
_____
_____

2. What's one thing you can do to make today great?

_____

Day: _____   Date: __/__/___

1. Today I am *Grateful* for:

_____
_____
_____
_____
_____

2. What's one thing you can do to make today great?

_____

Day: _____   Date: __/__/___

1. Today I am *Grateful* for:

_____
_____
_____
_____
_____

2. What's one thing you can do to make today great?

_____

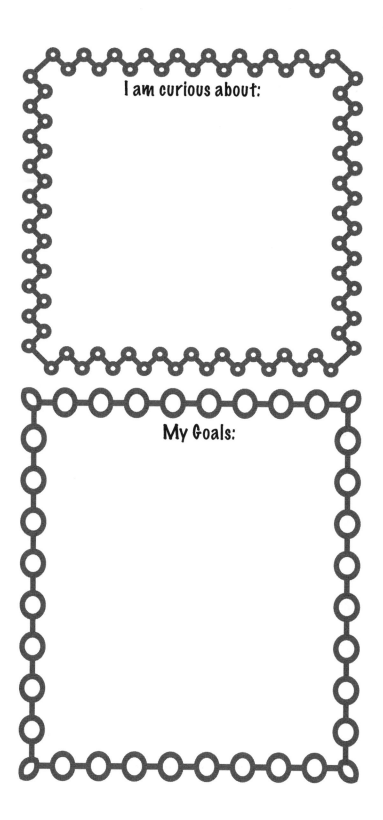

I am curious about:

My Goals:

To every action there is always opposed an equal reaction.
— Isaac Newton

Day: _____   Date: __/__/___

1. Today I am *Grateful* for:

_____

_____

_____

_____

_____

2. What's one thing you can do to make today great?

_____

Day: _____   Date: __/__/___

1. Today I am *Grateful* for:

_____

_____

_____

_____

_____

2. What's one thing you can do to make today great?

_____

Day: _____   Date: __/__/___

1. Today I am *Grateful* for:

_____

_____

_____

_____

_____

2. What's one thing you can do to make today great?

_____

When unhappy, one doubts everything; when happy, one
doubts nothing. — Joseph Roux

Day: _____   Date: __/__/___

1. Today I am *Grateful* for:

_____

_____

_____

_____

_____

2. What's one thing you can do to make today great?

_____

Day: _____   Date: __/__/___

1. Today I am *Grateful* for:

_____

_____

_____

_____

_____

2. What's one thing you can do to make today great?

_____

Day: _____   Date: __/__/___

1. Today I am *Grateful* for:

_____

_____

_____

_____

_____

2. What's one thing you can do to make today great?

_____

The harder the conflict, the more glorious the triumph.
— Thomas Paine

Day: _____   Date: __/__/___

1. Today I am *Grateful* for:

_____

_____

_____

_____

_____

2. What's one thing you can do to make today great?

_____

Day: _____   Date: __/__/___

1. Today I am *Grateful* for:

_____

_____

_____

_____

_____

2. What's one thing you can do to make today great?

_____

Day: _____   Date: __/__/___

1. Today I am *Grateful* for:

_____

_____

_____

_____

_____

2. What's one thing you can do to make today great?

_____

The soul that sees beauty may sometimes walk alone.
— Johann Wolfgang von Goethe

Day: _____   Date: __/__/___

1. Today I am *Grateful* for:

_____

_____

_____

_____

_____

2. What's one thing you can do to make today great?

_____

Day: _____   Date: __/__/___

1. Today I am *Grateful* for:

_____

_____

_____

_____

_____

2. What's one thing you can do to make today great?

_____

Day: _____   Date: __/__/___

1. Today I am *Grateful* for:

_____

_____

_____

_____

_____

2. What's one thing you can do to make today great?

_____

Tears of joy are like the summer rain drops pierced by sunbeams.
— Hosea Ballou

Day: _____   Date: __/__/___

1. Today I am *Grateful* for:

_____

_____

_____

_____

_____

2. What's one thing you can do to make today great?

_____

Day: _____   Date: __/__/___

1. Today I am *Grateful* for:

_____

_____

_____

_____

_____

2. What's one thing you can do to make today great?

_____

Day: _____   Date: __/__/___

1. Today I am *Grateful* for:

_____

_____

_____

_____

_____

2. What's one thing you can do to make today great?

_____

Everything that happens happens as it should, and if you observe
carefully, you will find this to be so. — Marcus Aurelius

Day: _____   Date: __/__/____

1. Today I am *Grateful* for:

_____

_____

_____

_____

_____

2. What's one thing you can do to make today great?

_____

Day: _____   Date: __/__/____

1. Today I am *Grateful* for:

_____

_____

_____

_____

_____

2. What's one thing you can do to make today great?

_____

Day: _____   Date: __/__/____

1. Today I am *Grateful* for:

_____

_____

_____

_____

_____

2. What's one thing you can do to make today great?

_____

The power of imagination makes us infinite.
— John Muir

Day: _____   Date: __/__/____

1. Today I am *Grateful* for:

_____
_____
_____
_____
_____

2. What's one thing you can do to make today great?

_____

Day: _____   Date: __/__/____

1. Today I am *Grateful* for:

_____
_____
_____
_____
_____

2. What's one thing you can do to make today great?

_____

Day: _____   Date: __/__/____

1. Today I am *Grateful* for:

_____
_____
_____
_____
_____

2. What's one thing you can do to make today great?

_____

Saying and doing are two things.
— Matthew Henry

Day: _____   Date: __/__/____

1. Today I am *Grateful* for:

_____

_____

_____

_____

_____

2. What's one thing you can do to make today great?

_____

Day: _____   Date: __/__/____

1. Today I am *Grateful* for:

_____

_____

_____

_____

_____

2. What's one thing you can do to make today great?

_____

Day: _____   Date: __/__/____

1. Today I am *Grateful* for:

_____

_____

_____

_____

_____

2. What's one thing you can do to make today great?

_____

To forget oneself is to be happy.
— Robert Louis Stevenson

Day: _____   Date: __/__/____

1. Today I am *Grateful* for:

_____

_____

_____

_____

_____

2. What's one thing you can do to make today great?

_____

Day: _____   Date: __/__/____

1. Today I am *Grateful* for:

_____

_____

_____

_____

2. What's one thing you can do to make today great?

_____

Day: _____   Date: __/__/____

1. Today I am *Grateful* for:

_____

_____

_____

_____

2. What's one thing you can do to make today great?

_____

When I let go of what I am, I become what I might be.
— Lao Tzu

Day: _____ 							Date: __/__/____

1. Today I am *Grateful* for:

_____

_____

_____

_____

_____

2. What's one thing you can do to make today great?

_____

Day: _____ 							Date: __/__/____

1. Today I am *Grateful* for:

_____

_____

_____

_____

_____

2. What's one thing you can do to make today great?

_____

Day: _____ 							Date: __/__/____

1. Today I am *Grateful* for:

_____

_____

_____

_____

_____

2. What's one thing you can do to make today great?

_____

A thousand words will not leave so deep an impression
as one deed. — Henrik Ibsen

Day: _____   Date: __/__/___

1. Today I am *Grateful* for:

_____

_____

_____

_____

_____

2. What's one thing you can do to make today great?

_____

Day: _____   Date: __/__/___

1. Today I am *Grateful* for:

_____

_____

_____

_____

_____

2. What's one thing you can do to make today great?

_____

Day: _____   Date: __/__/___

1. Today I am *Grateful* for:

_____

_____

_____

_____

_____

2. What's one thing you can do to make today great?

_____

Happiness depends upon ourselves.
— Aristotle

Day: _____   Date: __/__/____

1. Today I am *Grateful* for:

_____

_____

_____

_____

_____

2. What's one thing you can do to make today great?

_____

Day: _____   Date: __/__/____

1. Today I am *Grateful* for:

_____

_____

_____

_____

_____

2. What's one thing you can do to make today great?

_____

Day: _____   Date: __/__/____

1. Today I am *Grateful* for:

_____

_____

_____

_____

_____

2. What's one thing you can do to make today great?

_____

Day: _____   Date: __/__/___

1. Today I am *Grateful* for:

_____

_____

_____

_____

_____

_____

2. What's one thing you can do to make today great?

_____

Day: _____   Date: __/__/___

1. Today I am *Grateful* for:

_____

_____

_____

_____

_____

2. What's one thing you can do to make today great?

_____

Day: _____   Date: __/__/___

1. Today I am *Grateful* for:

_____

_____

_____

_____

_____

2. What's one thing you can do to make today great?

_____

In every walk with nature one receives far more than he seeks.
— John Muir

Day: _____   Date: __/__/____

1. Today I am *Grateful* for:

_____

_____

_____

_____

_____

_____

2. What's one thing you can do to make today great?

_____

Day: _____   Date: __/__/____

1. Today I am *Grateful* for:

_____

_____

_____

_____

_____

_____

2. What's one thing you can do to make today great?

_____

Day: _____   Date: __/__/____

1. Today I am *Grateful* for:

_____

_____

_____

_____

_____

_____

2. What's one thing you can do to make today great?

_____

What are my limiting beliefs?

What are my empowering beliefs?

The pursuit, even of the best things, ought to be calm
and tranquil. — Marcus Tullius Cicero

Day: _____   Date: __/__/____

1. Today I am *Grateful* for:

_____

_____

_____

_____

_____

2. What's one thing you can do to make today great?

_____

Day: _____   Date: __/__/____

1. Today I am *Grateful* for:

_____

_____

_____

_____

_____

2. What's one thing you can do to make today great?

_____

Day: _____   Date: __/__/____

1. Today I am *Grateful* for:

_____

_____

_____

_____

_____

2. What's one thing you can do to make today great?

_____

You never know what is enough unless you know what is more than enough. — William Blake

Day: _____   Date: __/__/____

1. Today I am *Grateful* for:

_____

_____

_____

_____

_____

2. What's one thing you can do to make today great?

_____

Day: _____   Date: __/__/____

1. Today I am *Grateful* for:

_____

_____

_____

_____

_____

2. What's one thing you can do to make today great?

_____

Day: _____   Date: __/__/____

1. Today I am *Grateful* for:

_____

_____

_____

_____

_____

2. What's one thing you can do to make today great?

_____

Fortune favors the bold.
— Virgil

Day: _____   Date: __/__/____

1. Today I am *Grateful* for:

_____

_____

_____

_____

_____

_____

2. What's one thing you can do to make today great?

_____

Day: _____   Date: __/__/____

1. Today I am *Grateful* for:

_____

_____

_____

_____

_____

_____

2. What's one thing you can do to make today great?

_____

Day: _____   Date: __/__/____

1. Today I am *Grateful* for:

_____

_____

_____

_____

_____

_____

2. What's one thing you can do to make today great?

_____

It is beyond a doubt that all our knowledge begins
with experience. — Immanuel Kant

Day: _____   Date: __/__/____

1. Today I am *Grateful* for:

_____

_____

_____

_____

_____

2. What's one thing you can do to make today great?

_____

Day: _____   Date: __/__/____

1. Today I am *Grateful* for:

_____

_____

_____

_____

_____

2. What's one thing you can do to make today great?

_____

Day: _____   Date: __/__/____

1. Today I am *Grateful* for:

_____

_____

_____

_____

_____

2. What's one thing you can do to make today great?

_____

Wisdom begins in wonder.
— Socrates

Day: _____   Date: __/__/____

1. Today I am *Grateful* for:

_____

_____

_____

_____

_____

2. What's one thing you can do to make today great?

_____

Day: _____   Date: __/__/____

1. Today I am *Grateful* for:

_____

_____

_____

_____

_____

2. What's one thing you can do to make today great?

_____

Day: _____   Date: __/__/____

1. Today I am *Grateful* for:

_____

_____

_____

_____

_____

2. What's one thing you can do to make today great?

_____

We love life, not because we are used to living but because
we are used to loving. — Friedrich Nietzsche

Day: _____   Date: _/_/___

1. Today I am *Grateful* for:

_____
_____
_____
_____
_____
_____

2. What's one thing you can do to make today great?

_____

Day: _____   Date: _/_/___

1. Today I am *Grateful* for:

_____
_____
_____
_____
_____
_____

2. What's one thing you can do to make today great?

_____

Day: _____   Date: _/_/___

1. Today I am *Grateful* for:

_____
_____
_____
_____
_____
_____

2. What's one thing you can do to make today great?

_____

Happiness is a virtue, not its reward.
— Baruch Spinoza

Day: _____   Date: __/__/____

1. Today I am *Grateful* for:

_____

_____

_____

_____

_____

_____

2. What's one thing you can do to make today great?

_____

Day: _____   Date: __/__/____

1. Today I am *Grateful* for:

_____

_____

_____

_____

_____

_____

2. What's one thing you can do to make today great?

_____

Day: _____   Date: __/__/____

1. Today I am *Grateful* for:

_____

_____

_____

_____

_____

2. What's one thing you can do to make today great?

_____

Success is sweet and sweeter if long delayed and gotten through many struggles and defeats. — Amos Bronson Alcott

Day: _____   Date: __/__/___

1. Today I am *Grateful* for:

_____

_____

_____

_____

_____

2. What's one thing you can do to make today great?

_____

Day: _____   Date: __/__/___

1. Today I am *Grateful* for:

_____

_____

_____

_____

_____

2. What's one thing you can do to make today great?

_____

Day: _____   Date: __/__/___

1. Today I am *Grateful* for:

_____

_____

_____

_____

_____

2. What's one thing you can do to make today great?

_____

A picture is a poem without words.
— Horace

Day: _____   Date: __/__/____

1. Today I am *Grateful* for:

_____

_____

_____

_____

_____

_____

2. What's one thing you can do to make today great?

_____

Day: _____   Date: __/__/____

1. Today I am *Grateful* for:

_____

_____

_____

_____

_____

_____

2. What's one thing you can do to make today great?

_____

Day: _____   Date: __/__/____

1. Today I am *Grateful* for:

_____

_____

_____

_____

_____

2. What's one thing you can do to make today great?

_____

Happiness is a choice that requires effort at times.
— Aeschylus

Day: _____   Date: _/_/___

1. Today I am *Grateful* for:

_____

_____

_____

_____

_____

2. What's one thing you can do to make today great?

_____

Day: _____   Date: _/_/___

1. Today I am *Grateful* for:

_____

_____

_____

_____

_____

2. What's one thing you can do to make today great?

_____

Day: _____   Date: _/_/___

1. Today I am *Grateful* for:

_____

_____

_____

_____

_____

2. What's one thing you can do to make today great?

_____

When words leave off, music begins.
— Heinrich Heine

Day: _____   Date: __/__/____

1. Today I am *Grateful* for:

_____

_____

_____

_____

_____

2. What's one thing you can do to make today great?

_____

Day: _____   Date: __/__/____

1. Today I am *Grateful* for:

_____

_____

_____

_____

_____

2. What's one thing you can do to make today great?

_____

Day: _____   Date: __/__/____

1. Today I am *Grateful* for:

_____

_____

_____

_____

_____

2. What's one thing you can do to make today great?

_____

There are two ways of spreading light: to be the candle or the mirror that reflects it. — Edith Wharton

Day: _____   Date: __/__/____

1. Today I am *Grateful* for:

_____

_____

_____

_____

_____

_____

2. What's one thing you can do to make today great?

_____

Day: _____   Date: __/__/____

1. Today I am *Grateful* for:

_____

_____

_____

_____

_____

_____

2. What's one thing you can do to make today great?

_____

Day: _____   Date: __/__/____

1. Today I am *Grateful* for:

_____

_____

_____

_____

_____

_____

2. What's one thing you can do to make today great?

_____

Nothing ever becomes real till it is experienced.
— John Keats

Day: _____   Date: __/__/___

1. Today I am *Grateful* for:

_____

_____

_____

_____

_____

_____

2. What's one thing you can do to make today great?

_____

Day: _____   Date: __/__/___

1. Today I am *Grateful* for:

_____

_____

_____

_____

_____

_____

2. What's one thing you can do to make today great?

_____

Day: _____   Date: __/__/___

1. Today I am *Grateful* for:

_____

_____

_____

_____

_____

_____

2. What's one thing you can do to make today great?

_____

If it were not for hopes, the heart would break.
— Thomas Fuller

Day: _____   Date: __/__/____

1. Today I am *Grateful* for:

_____

_____

_____

_____

_____

2. What's one thing you can do to make today great?

_____

Day: _____   Date: __/__/____

1. Today I am *Grateful* for:

_____

_____

_____

_____

_____

2. What's one thing you can do to make today great?

_____

Day: _____   Date: __/__/____

1. Today I am *Grateful* for:

_____

_____

_____

_____

_____

2. What's one thing you can do to make today great?

_____

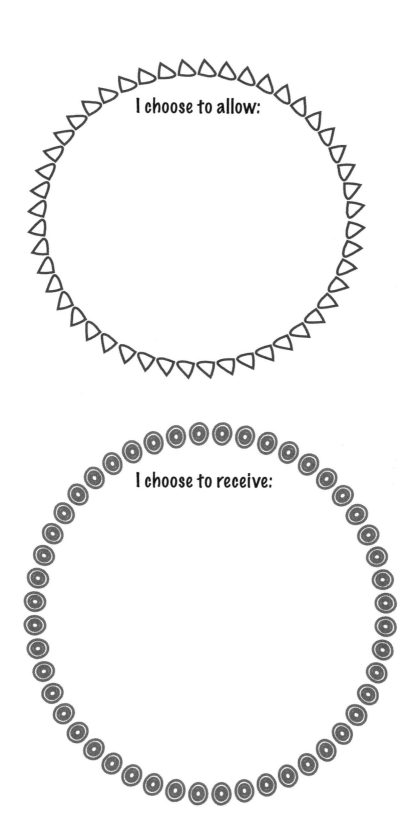

I choose to allow:

I choose to receive:

The things that we love tell us what we are.
— Thomas Aquinas

Day: _____   Date: __/__/____

1. Today I am *Grateful* for:

_____

_____

_____

_____

_____

2. What's one thing you can do to make today great?

_____

Day: _____   Date: __/__/____

1. Today I am *Grateful* for:

_____

_____

_____

_____

_____

2. What's one thing you can do to make today great?

_____

Day: _____   Date: __/__/____

1. Today I am *Grateful* for:

_____

_____

_____

_____

_____

2. What's one thing you can do to make today great?

_____

Keep your face always toward the sunshine - and shadows
will fall behind you. — Walt Whitman

Day: _____   Date: _/_/___

1. Today I am *Grateful* for:

_____

_____

_____

_____

_____

_____

2. What's one thing you can do to make today great?

_____

Day: _____   Date: _/_/___

1. Today I am *Grateful* for:

_____

_____

_____

_____

_____

2. What's one thing you can do to make today great?

_____

Day: _____   Date: _/_/___

1. Today I am *Grateful* for:

_____

_____

_____

_____

_____

2. What's one thing you can do to make today great?

_____

To the artist there is never anything ugly in nature.
— Auguste Rodin

Day: _____   Date: __/__/____

1. Today I am *Grateful* for:

_____

_____

_____

_____

_____

2. What's one thing you can do to make today great?

_____

Day: _____   Date: __/__/____

1. Today I am *Grateful* for:

_____

_____

_____

_____

_____

2. What's one thing you can do to make today great?

_____

Day: _____   Date: __/__/____

1. Today I am *Grateful* for:

_____

_____

_____

_____

_____

2. What's one thing you can do to make today great?

_____

One must still have chaos in oneself to be able to give birth
to a dancing star. — Friedrich Nietzsche

Day: _____   Date: __/__/____

1. Today I am *Grateful* for:

_____

_____

_____

_____

_____

2. What's one thing you can do to make today great?

_____

Day: _____   Date: __/__/____

1. Today I am *Grateful* for:

_____

_____

_____

_____

_____

2. What's one thing you can do to make today great?

_____

Day: _____   Date: __/__/____

1. Today I am *Grateful* for:

_____

_____

_____

_____

_____

2. What's one thing you can do to make today great?

_____

To live is so startling it leaves little time for anything else.
— Emily Dickinson

Day: _____   Date: __/__/____

1. Today I am *Grateful* for:

_____
_____
_____
_____
_____

2. What's one thing you can do to make today great?

_____

Day: _____   Date: __/__/____

1. Today I am *Grateful* for:

_____
_____
_____
_____
_____

2. What's one thing you can do to make today great?

_____

Day: _____   Date: __/__/____

1. Today I am *Grateful* for:

_____
_____
_____
_____
_____

2. What's one thing you can do to make today great?

_____

That man is a success who has lived well, laughed
often and loved much. — Robert Louis Stevenson

Day: _____   Date: __/__/____

1. Today I am *Grateful* for:

_____

_____

_____

_____

_____

2. What's one thing you can do to make today great?

_____

Day: _____   Date: __/__/____

1. Today I am *Grateful* for:

_____

_____

_____

_____

_____

2. What's one thing you can do to make today great?

_____

Day: _____   Date: __/__/____

1. Today I am *Grateful* for:

_____

_____

_____

_____

_____

2. What's one thing you can do to make today great?

_____

Positive anything is better than negative nothing.
— Elbert Hubbard

Day: _____   Date: __/__/____

1. Today I am *Grateful* for:

_____

_____

_____

_____

_____

_____

2. What's one thing you can do to make today great?

_____

Day: _____   Date: __/__/____

1. Today I am *Grateful* for:

_____

_____

_____

_____

_____

_____

2. What's one thing you can do to make today great?

_____

Day: _____   Date: __/__/____

1. Today I am *Grateful* for:

_____

_____

_____

_____

_____

_____

2. What's one thing you can do to make today great?

_____

No act of kindness, no matter how small, is ever wasted.
— Aesop

Day: _____   Date: __/__/____

1. Today I am *Grateful* for:

_____

_____

_____

_____

_____

2. What's one thing you can do to make today great?

_____

Day: _____   Date: __/__/____

1. Today I am *Grateful* for:

_____

_____

_____

_____

_____

2. What's one thing you can do to make today great?

_____

Day: _____   Date: __/__/____

1. Today I am *Grateful* for:

_____

_____

_____

_____

_____

2. What's one thing you can do to make today great?

_____

Creativity is not the finding of a thing, but the making something out of it after it is found. — James Russell Lowell

Day: _____   Date: __/__/____

1. Today I am *Grateful* for:

_____

_____

_____

_____

_____

2. What's one thing you can do to make today great?

_____

Day: _____   Date: __/__/____

1. Today I am *Grateful* for:

_____

_____

_____

_____

_____

2. What's one thing you can do to make today great?

_____

Day: _____   Date: __/__/____

1. Today I am *Grateful* for:

_____

_____

_____

_____

_____

2. What's one thing you can do to make today great?

_____

Wonder is the desire for knowledge.
— Thomas Aquinas

Day: _____   Date: __/__/____

1. Today I am *Grateful* for:

_____

_____

_____

_____

_____

2. What's one thing you can do to make today great?

_____

Day: _____   Date: __/__/____

1. Today I am *Grateful* for:

_____

_____

_____

_____

_____

2. What's one thing you can do to make today great?

_____

Day: _____   Date: __/__/____

1. Today I am *Grateful* for:

_____

_____

_____

_____

_____

2. What's one thing you can do to make today great?

_____

The way to know life is to love many things.
— Vincent Van Gogh

Day: _____   Date: __/__/___

1. Today I am *Grateful* for:

_____

_____

_____

_____

_____

2. What's one thing you can do to make today great?

_____

Day: _____   Date: __/__/___

1. Today I am *Grateful* for:

_____

_____

_____

_____

_____

2. What's one thing you can do to make today great?

_____

Day: _____   Date: __/__/___

1. Today I am *Grateful* for:

_____

_____

_____

_____

_____

2. What's one thing you can do to make today great?

_____

We cannot wish for that we know not.
— Voltaire

Day: _____   Date: __/__/____

1. Today I am *Grateful* for:

_____

_____

_____

_____

_____

2. What's one thing you can do to make today great?

_____

Day: _____   Date: __/__/____

1. Today I am *Grateful* for:

_____

_____

_____

_____

_____

2. What's one thing you can do to make today great?

_____

Day: _____   Date: __/__/____

1. Today I am *Grateful* for:

_____

_____

_____

_____

_____

2. What's one thing you can do to make today great?

_____

To begin, begin.
— William Wordsworth

Day: _____   Date: __/__/____

1. Today I am *Grateful* for:

_____

_____

_____

_____

_____

2. What's one thing you can do to make today great?

_____

Day: _____   Date: __/__/____

1. Today I am *Grateful* for:

_____

_____

_____

_____

_____

2. What's one thing you can do to make today great?

_____

Day: _____   Date: __/__/____

1. Today I am *Grateful* for:

_____

_____

_____

_____

_____

2. What's one thing you can do to make today great?

_____

The greatest weapon against stress is our ability to
choose one thought over another. — William James

Day: _____   Date: __/__/____

1. Today I am *Grateful* for:

_____

_____

_____

_____

_____

2. What's one thing you can do to make today great?

_____

Day: _____   Date: __/__/____

1. Today I am *Grateful* for:

_____

_____

_____

_____

_____

2. What's one thing you can do to make today great?

_____

Day: _____   Date: __/__/____

1. Today I am *Grateful* for:

_____

_____

_____

_____

_____

2. What's one thing you can do to make today great?

_____

I am:

I affirm:

Success is dependent on effort.
— Sophocles

Day: _____   Date: __/__/____

1. Today I am *Grateful* for:

_____

_____

_____

_____

_____

2. What's one thing you can do to make today great?

_____

Day: _____   Date: __/__/____

1. Today I am *Grateful* for:

_____

_____

_____

_____

_____

2. What's one thing you can do to make today great?

_____

Day: _____   Date: __/__/____

1. Today I am *Grateful* for:

_____

_____

_____

_____

_____

2. What's one thing you can do to make today great?

_____

There are lots of people who mistake their imagination
for their memory. — Josh Billings

Day: _____   Date: __/__/____

1. Today I am *Grateful* for:

_____

_____

_____

_____

_____

2. What's one thing you can do to make today great?

_____

Day: _____   Date: __/__/____

1. Today I am *Grateful* for:

_____

_____

_____

_____

_____

2. What's one thing you can do to make today great?

_____

Day: _____   Date: __/__/____

1. Today I am *Grateful* for:

_____

_____

_____

_____

_____

2. What's one thing you can do to make today great?

_____

We are here to add what we can to life, not to get what
we can from life. — William Osler

Day: _____   Date: __/__/___

1. Today I am *Grateful* for:

_____

_____

_____

_____

_____

2. What's one thing you can do to make today great?

_____

Day: _____   Date: __/__/___

1. Today I am *Grateful* for:

_____

_____

_____

_____

_____

2. What's one thing you can do to make today great?

_____

Day: _____   Date: __/__/___

1. Today I am *Grateful* for:

_____

_____

_____

_____

_____

2. What's one thing you can do to make today great?

_____

All experience is an arch, to build upon.
— Henry Adams

Day: _____   Date: __/__/____

1. Today I am *Grateful* for:

_____

_____

_____

_____

_____

2. What's one thing you can do to make today great?

_____

Day: _____   Date: __/__/____

1. Today I am *Grateful* for:

_____

_____

_____

_____

_____

2. What's one thing you can do to make today great?

_____

Day: _____   Date: __/__/____

1. Today I am *Grateful* for:

_____

_____

_____

_____

_____

2. What's one thing you can do to make today great?

_____

Be not simply good - be good for something.
— Henry David Thoreau

Day: _____   Date: __/__/____

1. Today I am *Grateful* for:

_____

_____

_____

_____

_____

2. What's one thing you can do to make today great?

_____

Day: _____   Date: __/__/____

1. Today I am *Grateful* for:

_____

_____

_____

_____

_____

2. What's one thing you can do to make today great?

_____

Day: _____   Date: __/__/____

1. Today I am *Grateful* for:

_____

_____

_____

_____

_____

2. What's one thing you can do to make today great?

_____

The best thinking has been done in solitude. The worst has been done in turmoil. — Thomas A. Edison

Day: _____   Date: __/__/____

1. Today I am *Grateful* for:

_____

_____

_____

_____

_____

2. What's one thing you can do to make today great?

_____

Day: _____   Date: __/__/____

1. Today I am *Grateful* for:

_____

_____

_____

_____

_____

2. What's one thing you can do to make today great?

_____

Day: _____   Date: __/__/____

1. Today I am *Grateful* for:

_____

_____

_____

_____

_____

2. What's one thing you can do to make today great?

_____

Be as you wish to seem.
— Socrates

Day: _____   Date: __/__/____

1. Today I am *Grateful* for:

_____
_____
_____
_____
_____

2. What's one thing you can do to make today great?

_____

Day: _____   Date: __/__/____

1. Today I am *Grateful* for:

_____
_____
_____
_____
_____

2. What's one thing you can do to make today great?

_____

Day: _____   Date: __/__/____

1. Today I am *Grateful* for:

_____
_____
_____
_____

2. What's one thing you can do to make today great?

_____

Persevere and preserve yourselves for better circumstances.
— Virgil

Day: _____   Date: _/_/___

1. Today I am *Grateful* for:

_____

_____

_____

_____

_____

_____

2. What's one thing you can do to make today great?

_____

Day: _____   Date: _/_/___

1. Today I am *Grateful* for:

_____

_____

_____

_____

_____

2. What's one thing you can do to make today great?

_____

Day: _____   Date: _/_/___

1. Today I am *Grateful* for:

_____

_____

_____

_____

_____

2. What's one thing you can do to make today great?

_____

Life is the flower for which love is the honey.
— Victor Hugo

Day: _____   Date: __/__/____

1. Today I am *Grateful* for:

_____

_____

_____

_____

_____

2. What's one thing you can do to make today great?

_____

Day: _____   Date: __/__/____

1. Today I am *Grateful* for:

_____

_____

_____

_____

_____

2. What's one thing you can do to make today great?

_____

Day: _____   Date: __/__/____

1. Today I am *Grateful* for:

_____

_____

_____

_____

_____

2. What's one thing you can do to make today great?

_____

Every noble work is at first impossible.
— Thomas Carlyle

Day: _____   Date: __/__/____

1. Today I am *Grateful* for:

_____
_____
_____
_____
_____
_____

2. What's one thing you can do to make today great?

_____

Day: _____   Date: __/__/____

1. Today I am *Grateful* for:

_____
_____
_____
_____
_____
_____

2. What's one thing you can do to make today great?

_____

Day: _____   Date: __/__/____

1. Today I am *Grateful* for:

_____
_____
_____
_____
_____
_____

2. What's one thing you can do to make today great?

_____

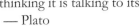

Day: _____   Date: __/__/____

1. Today I am *Grateful* for:

_____

_____

_____

_____

_____

2. What's one thing you can do to make today great?

_____

Day: _____   Date: __/__/____

1. Today I am *Grateful* for:

_____

_____

_____

_____

_____

2. What's one thing you can do to make today great?

_____

Day: _____   Date: __/__/____

1. Today I am *Grateful* for:

_____

_____

_____

_____

_____

2. What's one thing you can do to make today great?

_____

Painting from nature is not copying the object; it is realizing one's sensations. — Paul Cezanne

Day: _____   Date: __/__/____

1. Today I am *Grateful* for:

_____

_____

_____

_____

_____

2. What's one thing you can do to make today great?

_____

Day: _____   Date: __/__/____

1. Today I am *Grateful* for:

_____

_____

_____

_____

_____

2. What's one thing you can do to make today great?

_____

Day: _____   Date: __/__/____

1. Today I am *Grateful* for:

_____

_____

_____

_____

_____

2. What's one thing you can do to make today great?

_____

Tenderness is a virtue.
— Oliver Goldsmith

Day: _____   Date: __/__/____

1. Today I am *Grateful* for:

_____

_____

_____

_____

_____

_____

2. What's one thing you can do to make today great?

_____

Day: _____   Date: __/__/____

1. Today I am *Grateful* for:

_____

_____

_____

_____

_____

_____

2. What's one thing you can do to make today great?

_____

Day: _____   Date: __/__/____

1. Today I am *Grateful* for:

_____

_____

_____

_____

_____

2. What's one thing you can do to make today great?

_____

Imagination is the eye of the soul.
— Joseph Joubert

Day: _____   Date: __/__/___

1. Today I am *Grateful* for:

_____

_____

_____

_____

_____

_____

2. What's one thing you can do to make today great?

_____

Day: _____   Date: __/__/___

1. Today I am *Grateful* for:

_____

_____

_____

_____

_____

_____

2. What's one thing you can do to make today great?

_____

Day: _____   Date: __/__/___

1. Today I am *Grateful* for:

_____

_____

_____

_____

_____

_____

2. What's one thing you can do to make today great?

_____

What's on your mind?

What do you want?

Why do you want it?

I hear and I forget. I see and I remember. I do and
I understand. — Confucius

Day: _____   Date: __/__/___

1. Today I am *Grateful* for:

_____

_____

_____

_____

_____

2. What's one thing you can do to make today great?

_____

Day: _____   Date: __/__/___

1. Today I am *Grateful* for:

_____

_____

_____

_____

_____

2. What's one thing you can do to make today great?

_____

Day: _____   Date: __/__/___

1. Today I am *Grateful* for:

_____

_____

_____

_____

_____

2. What's one thing you can do to make today great?

_____

What worries you, masters you.
— John Locke

Day: _____   Date: _/_/___

1. Today I am *Grateful* for:

_____

_____

_____

_____

_____

2. What's one thing you can do to make today great?

_____

Day: _____   Date: _/_/___

1. Today I am *Grateful* for:

_____

_____

_____

_____

_____

2. What's one thing you can do to make today great?

_____

Day: _____   Date: _/_/___

1. Today I am *Grateful* for:

_____

_____

_____

_____

_____

2. What's one thing you can do to make today great?

_____

This world is but a canvas to our imagination.
— Henry David Thoreau

Day: _____   Date: __/__/____

1. Today I am *Grateful* for:

_____

_____

_____

_____

_____

2. What's one thing you can do to make today great?

_____

Day: _____   Date: __/__/____

1. Today I am *Grateful* for:

_____

_____

_____

_____

_____

2. What's one thing you can do to make today great?

_____

Day: _____   Date: __/__/____

1. Today I am *Grateful* for:

_____

_____

_____

_____

_____

2. What's one thing you can do to make today great?

_____

Let the beauty of what you love be what you do.
— Rumi

Day: _____   Date: __/__/____

1. Today I am *Grateful* for:

_____

_____

_____

_____

_____

2. What's one thing you can do to make today great?

_____

Day: _____   Date: __/__/____

1. Today I am *Grateful* for:

_____

_____

_____

_____

_____

2. What's one thing you can do to make today great?

_____

Day: _____   Date: __/__/____

1. Today I am *Grateful* for:

_____

_____

_____

_____

_____

2. What's one thing you can do to make today great?

_____

There is nothing like a dream to create the future.
— Victor Hugo

Day: _____   Date: __/__/____

1. Today I am *Grateful* for:

_____

_____

_____

_____

_____

2. What's one thing you can do to make today great?

_____

Day: _____   Date: __/__/____

1. Today I am *Grateful* for:

_____

_____

_____

_____

_____

2. What's one thing you can do to make today great?

_____

Day: _____   Date: __/__/____

1. Today I am *Grateful* for:

_____

_____

_____

_____

_____

2. What's one thing you can do to make today great?

_____

You cannot do a kindness too soon, for you never know
how soon it will be too late. — Ralph Waldo Emerson

Day: _____   Date: __/__/____

1. Today I am *Grateful* for:

_____

_____

_____

_____

_____

2. What's one thing you can do to make today great?

_____

Day: _____   Date: __/__/____

1. Today I am *Grateful* for:

_____

_____

_____

_____

_____

2. What's one thing you can do to make today great?

_____

Day: _____   Date: __/__/____

1. Today I am *Grateful* for:

_____

_____

_____

_____

_____

2. What's one thing you can do to make today great?

_____

A single grateful thought toward heaven is the most perfect prayer.
— Gotthold Ephraim Lessing

Day: _____   Date: __/__/____

1. Today I am *Grateful* for:

_____

_____

_____

_____

_____

2. What's one thing you can do to make today great?

_____

Day: _____   Date: __/__/____

1. Today I am *Grateful* for:

_____

_____

_____

_____

_____

2. What's one thing you can do to make today great?

_____

Day: _____   Date: __/__/____

1. Today I am *Grateful* for:

_____

_____

_____

_____

_____

2. What's one thing you can do to make today great?

_____

The real voyage of discovery consists not in seeking new landscapes, but in having new eyes. — Marcel Proust

Day: _____   Date: __/__/____

1. Today I am *Grateful* for:

_____

_____

_____

_____

_____

2. What's one thing you can do to make today great?

_____

Day: _____   Date: __/__/____

1. Today I am *Grateful* for:

_____

_____

_____

_____

_____

2. What's one thing you can do to make today great?

_____

Day: _____   Date: __/__/____

1. Today I am *Grateful* for:

_____

_____

_____

_____

_____

2. What's one thing you can do to make today great?

_____

Never give up, for that is just the place and time
that the tide will turn. — Harriet Beecher Stowe

Day: _____   Date: __/__/____

1. Today I am *Grateful* for:

_____

_____

_____

_____

_____

2. What's one thing you can do to make today great?

_____

Day: _____   Date: __/__/____

1. Today I am *Grateful* for:

_____

_____

_____

_____

_____

2. What's one thing you can do to make today great?

_____

Day: _____   Date: __/__/____

1. Today I am *Grateful* for:

_____

_____

_____

_____

_____

2. What's one thing you can do to make today great?

_____

The best thing one can do when it's raining is to let it rain.
— Henry Wadsworth Longfellow

Day: _____   Date: _/_/____

1. Today I am *Grateful* for:

_____

_____

_____

_____

_____

2. What's one thing you can do to make today great?

_____

Day: _____   Date: _/_/____

1. Today I am *Grateful* for:

_____

_____

_____

_____

_____

2. What's one thing you can do to make today great?

_____

Day: _____   Date: _/_/____

1. Today I am *Grateful* for:

_____

_____

_____

_____

_____

2. What's one thing you can do to make today great?

_____

The risk of a wrong decision is preferable to the
terror of indecision. — Maimonides

Day: _____   Date: __/__/____

1. Today I am *Grateful* for:

_____

_____

_____

_____

_____

_____

2. What's one thing you can do to make today great?

_____

Day: _____   Date: __/__/____

1. Today I am *Grateful* for:

_____

_____

_____

_____

_____

_____

2. What's one thing you can do to make today great?

_____

Day: _____   Date: __/__/____

1. Today I am *Grateful* for:

_____

_____

_____

_____

_____

2. What's one thing you can do to make today great?

_____

A gentle word, a kind look, a good-natured smile can work
wonders and accomplish miracles. — William Hazlitt

Day: _____   Date: __/__/____

1. Today I am *Grateful* for:

_____
_____
_____
_____
_____

2. What's one thing you can do to make today great?

_____

Day: _____   Date: __/__/____

1. Today I am *Grateful* for:

_____
_____
_____
_____
_____

2. What's one thing you can do to make today great?

_____

Day: _____   Date: __/__/____

1. Today I am *Grateful* for:

_____
_____
_____
_____
_____

2. What's one thing you can do to make today great?

_____

Do not take life too seriously. You will never get out of it alive.
— Elbert Hubbard

Day: _____   Date: __/__/____

1. Today I am *Grateful* for:

_____

_____

_____

_____

_____

2. What's one thing you can do to make today great?

_____

Day: _____   Date: __/__/____

1. Today I am *Grateful* for:

_____

_____

_____

_____

_____

2. What's one thing you can do to make today great?

_____

Day: _____   Date: __/__/____

1. Today I am *Grateful* for:

_____

_____

_____

_____

_____

2. What's one thing you can do to make today great?

_____

Without craftsmanship, inspiration is a mere reed shaken in the wind.
— Johannes Brahms

Day: _____   Date: __/__/____

1. Today I am *Grateful* for:

_____

_____

_____

_____

_____

2. What's one thing you can do to make today great?

_____

Day: _____   Date: __/__/____

1. Today I am *Grateful* for:

_____

_____

_____

_____

_____

2. What's one thing you can do to make today great?

_____

Day: _____   Date: __/__/____

1. Today I am *Grateful* for:

_____

_____

_____

_____

_____

2. What's one thing you can do to make today great?

_____

What does an extraordinary life look like for you?

Notes

Draw something

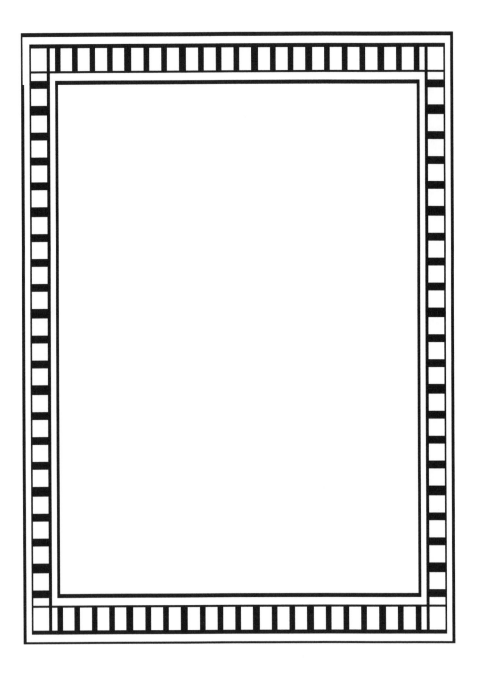